I0439760

Battling Ropes

Build Muscle, Lose Weight, Increase Strength & Endurance with Battling Rope Workouts

Table of Contents

Copyright

abuse of any policies, processes, or directions contained within is the solitary and utter responsibility of the recipient reader. Under no circumstances will any legal responsibility or blame be held against the publisher for any reparation, damages, or monetary loss due to the information herein, either directly or indirectly. Respective authors own all copyrights not held by the publisher.

The information herein is offered for informational purposes solely, and is universal as so. The presentation of the information is without contract or any type of guarantee assurance.

The trademarks that are used are without any consent, and the publication of the trademark is without permission or backing by the trademark owner. All trademarks and brands within this book are for clarifying purposes only and are the owned by the owners themselves, not affiliated with this document.

Introduction

This book will guide you in battling ropes usage to gain the amazing benefits of battle rope workouts that are often difficult to achieve through more conventional training tools.

Battle ropes are becoming very popular mainly due to the fact that they have specific advantages compared to most conventional tools; so much so that many famous athletes such as MMA fighters and Olympians are known to perform battle rope workouts.

Battle ropes workouts are naturally non-impact and dynamic physical training, which can be used for building muscle, losing weight, and increasing strength and endurance particularly by athletes. As a non-impact exercise, battle roping is ideal if you have problems in the bones or joints, or if you need to recover from an injury. Hence, there is less risk of injury compared to weight training.

Furthermore, battle ropes can offer immediate performance feedback, which is not possible. Conventional weight-training requires increasing weight to add difficulty and trigger muscle gains. However, the weights can only be added up in increments. Hence, there's no way to measure the force and speed. In contrast, the difficult in battle rope workouts can be created immediately and the feedback as to the production of force and speed can also be instant. The bigger and faster you create waves, the harder the movement is and hence you are exerting more force. Primary movers such as lats, quads, and shoulders can easily react by exerting effort to make bigger waves.

There are several training tools with particular advantage and will not cost you a hefty sum of money. All you need to do is to find a battle rope, tie it on a strong anchor and start working out to reap the rewards of a remarkable physical training.

Chapter 1- The Rules to Follow

The key to the effectiveness of battle workouts is that you need to work each arm separately, getting rid of imbalances in endurance as you gain muscles. It is important to follow the specific rules to maximize the benefits.

1. Use a standard battle rope
Battle ropes are available in different lengths and thicknesses. However, a 1-inch thick, 50-foot rope is recommended. You can even create your own battle rope. Just buy a generic rope (1.5 inch, 50 feet). Wrap the ends in duct tape, and anchor around a sturdy pole.

2. Move in Different Directions
It is ideal to try different movements to work out different muscle groups. For instance, moving from side to side will train your hips and core, which builds stability. Meanwhile, swinging the ropes in circular motion will minimize the risk of injury. Changing one type of motion to another will help you develop strong and lean muscles, and will also improve your body's flexibility and endurance.

3. Use Battle Ropes Regularly

Most guys use battle ropes as a workout finisher or as one component exercise in a bigger circuit. However, you can maximize the benefits if you choose to perform battle rope exercises more often. You can do most exercises described in this book for 10 to 15 minutes then perform waves alone for 20 minutes. Performing one task for longer duration will teach your mind to concentrate and help your body reduce lactic acid. This will also extend the time that your muscles will be under tension that will help you maximize strength as you try to lose fat.

4. Control the Resistance

The number of slow waves in the rope will measure the load. When you move away from the anchor point will reduce the intensity of the workout, while moving forward the anchor point will increase it. Control the resistance so you can vary the challenge in every set. If you are performing a battle rope workout, you can choose to do alternate exercises and at least two minutes away from the anchor. Take note that the time you spend away from the anchor is regarded as active recovery.

Chapter 2 – Building Muscle

Building muscle is possible as long as you know and apply the science of muscle growth, which is observable, repeatable, and certain. When you throw an apple up in the air, it will certainly come down. Once you perform the right actions in doing battle rope exercises, you will definitely grow muscles. It is really simple, and the science behind muscle growth is applicable regardless of your workout.

There are three primary hormones in the body that are important in growing strong and lean muscles. These are growth hormone, testosterone, and insulin growth factor-1. These three hormones work together to help the body develop muscles. So basically if you lack one hormone, it will be difficult to achieve a lean body that you want. For instance, testosterone boosts insulin growth factor but not without the growth hormone.

In order to build lean muscles, you need control these three hormones through training, nutrition and rest.

These muscle growth principles are known and followed for many years by athletes who have the best physique in the world. These laws are very practical. Once you follow them, you will see results. And once you feel and see your body getting leaner and bulkier, you will certainly believe that they're true.

Muscle Growth Law No. 1 - Muscles Grow only through Hard Work

You may say that this law is quite obvious and unnecessary to include in this book. However, many still don't get it. By doing battle rope exercises, you will cause tiny tears in the muscular tissues that the body will repair to strengthen muscles to better adapt to the stimulus that trigger the damage. This process is known as hypertrophy.

If the exercises cause very minimal tears in the muscle it is possible for muscle growth to happen because the body will be able to handle it. If the exercises cause too many muscle tears, then the body will not be able to repair the muscle tissues, and so muscle growth will not be possible. If the exercises cause enough muscle tear, but the body is not provided with enough rest and nutrition, muscle growth will not be possible.

For optimal muscle gain, you must perform battle ropes exercises in such a way that will cause enough muscle tears and you must be nourished and take enough rest.

Muscle Growth Law No. 2 - Overload Grows Muscle not Fatigue

While you may think that a burning sensation in the muscles is an indication of a beneficial workout, it don't actually indicate optimum workout. The sensation is caused by the infusion of lactic acid in the muscle that is produced as muscle burns stored energy. Lactic acid triggers release of growth-inducing hormones. However, increasing levels of lactic acid in the body will not guarantee more muscles.

Muscle fatigue is also not a sign of developing muscles. The sense of tiredness that you feel when you are training is an indication that blood is trapped in the muscles. Repetition is not enough to trigger muscle development. What you need is known as overload. Your muscular system should be given with clear reasons to develop, and that reason is overload. Some so called "experts" in muscle-gaining techniques would recommend performing different types of workouts. This is not true. You can develop muscle gains by doing the same mass-building workouts by steadily increasing your reps in the battle ropes to trigger overload.

Muscle Growth Law No. 3 - Muscles Develop After Workout

Conventional training programs will require you to train too often usually influenced by the usual misconception that muscle building is just a matter of excessive workout. If you have this bad habit, you need to realize that if you are doing less, you can get more. It is important to take note that muscles develop in between training the same muscle groups. Once you overload your muscles, your body can learn how to handle overloads. In order to grow muscles correctly, your body needs enough rest and nutrition.

If every day you are training the same muscle group, you will only lose your strength and not gain muscle size you want. If you let your muscles rest enough and eat properly, however, you will gain optimize both strength and muscle size.

Muscle Growth Law No. 4 - Muscles Grow If Your Body is Well Nourished

Nutrition is important in developing muscles. Your diet will determine your physique. You can perform the best battle rope workouts and get enough rest, but without proper nutrition, don't expect your muscles to grow.

Most athletes who do battling ropes exercises will get this wrong. They don't make sure that their body is getting its needs to easily grow muscle. Certainly, you have been told to eat proteins, but how much and when? What types of carbs should you take? When should you eat carbs to optimize muscle gain? Are fats essential in your battle rope regimen? How many calories should you take daily? It is crucial to know the answers for these questions if you want to maximize your battle ropes training for muscle gain.

Exercises to Optimize Muscle Gain

Power Slam

Stand with your feet apart and hold the rope in each hand. Raise both arms above your head and with all your power, slam down the ropes to the ground, doing a high squat. Straighten your body to stand and repeat. A variation of this is the alternate-arm, in which you need to perform the same movement, but instead of both hands slamming simultaneously, you need to hold the movement to only one arm. Perform alternating sets for each arm.

Slide Slam Alternating Waves

This battle rope exercise will sculpt your obliques. Hold the rope in each hand, and bent your knees slightly. Brace your core and hold the rope on the left. Raise your arms above your head and slam down the ropes to the right. Do alternating slams.

Knee Tuck Slams Alternating Waves

Get into a push-up position. Hold the rope in each hand and face the anchor. Jump with both feet in mid-air trying to move your knees toward your chest or knee tuck. Quickly go back into a push-up position, and then immediately jump with your feet at least a hip-width apart still holding on to the ropes. Raise both arms above your head and then try to flex your body until you are touching your toes. Go to a squat position, and then slam the rope down to the ground. Go back to push up position then do at least 10 repetitions.

You can kiss away bicep curls, calve raises, or sophisticated training machines. These trainings move muscle groups and will trigger better hormone response. By doing these important exercises, you can get more and avoid wasting energy.

Nutrition for muscle building

After a rigorous workout, you need to make certain that you are eating right to help your body recover for better muscle growth. The first thing you need to do is to take a week and record all the things you eat. Whether you munched in chocolate bar or veggies, log them. This will provide you a great idea on how much calories you are taking every day and every week.

Record everything you eat for at least one week, and check if you are gaining weight without being fat. If you are adding at least one pound every week and your body is still lean, you are doing good.

Be sure to add the following foods to your diet:

Beef

Beef is essential to build lean muscle because it is rich in protein, B vitamins, zinc, and iron. However, beef that are grass-fed are ideal as they have higher levels of conjugated linoleic acid or CLA that helps the body in reducing body fat.

Brown Rice

Brown rice is ideal than white rice because it takes longer to digest providing more energy throughout the day. Brown rice can also help in increasing growth hormone levels that are essential for fat loss and lean muscle gain.

Eggs

Eggs are regarded as the perfect protein. However, the muscle gain is not only due to the protein content. Cholesterol found in the egg yolks is also essential. If you are worried about too much cholesterol from eating egg yolks, research shows that the egg cholesterol combats the amount of bad cholesterol linked with atherosclerosis.

Beets

Beets are high in trimethylgycine that helps in enhancing liver and joint repair but also in developing muscle power and strength.

Other foods that can be added in your diet for lean muscle gain are oranges, cantaloupe, milk, quinoa, spinach, apples, and Greek yogurt.

It is important to take note that it will take some time to develop lean muscle gain. If you are adding at least 1 to 2 pounds per week, you are doing great. You can try getting a body fat test to make certain that what you are putting on are muscles and not fat. Be consistent with your training, nutrition, and rest.

Chapter 3 – Losing Weight with Battle Ropes Exercises

The human body has the ability to use different sources of energy during exercises. The first energy source is glycogen or carbohydrates that are stored in the muscle and liver. The second energy source is fat that is stored in adipose tissues and muscle as triglyceride.

However, the body's glycogen reserve is very limited, because it can only provide energy for high strenuous exercises such as battling ropes workouts. Once this energy reserve is depleted, the body will suffer from hypoglycemia that could lead to fatigue.

Meanwhile, fat storage is not often limited. An average human body has more than enough fat to sustain heavy workout, even in the case of athletes. Average people usually have surplus of fat storage, and so your objective in doing battle ropes exercises is to cut down on fat storage into an acceptable level.

Battle Rope Interval Training for Weight Loss

Before starting any kind of battle rope exercise, it is crucial that you understand first the benefits and value of doing High Intensity Interval Training or HIIT.

In general, HIIT is a basic method of training for people who want to lose weight or for athletes who want to get lean. HIIT is an efficient type of exercise that provides similar benefits in the long term. Basically, HIIT is nothing more than a method of training, which uses alternating periods of training and recuperation.

There are several physiological benefits of high intensity battle ropes exercises. This includes increased level of metabolic enzymes, increased muscle glycogen during rest period, better oxygen response after workout, better activity of respiratory and heart muscles, and better reduction of fat under the skin.

Battle Ropes Exercises for Weight Loss

Perform any three of battle ropes exercises below at least three times a week with one day rest period in between.

Reverse Lunge Alternating Wave

This battle rope exercise is great for the reduction of subcutaneous fat (fat under skin) not only for the upper body but also for the lower body focusing on the forearms, biceps, quadriceps, abs, and back. Start by doing basic wave steps. When you get a constant wave, lunge your right leg back. Stand again and then repeat for your left leg lunge. Continue alternating steps as you make waves with the battle ropes, keeping your chest and head straight up during the course of the workout.

Snakes Up and Downs

Stand firmly in the floor and hold the ropes in both hands, holding the ends at your side. Immediately drop your body to the ground and place your hands in a push-up position as you land on the floor. Allow your chest to touch the floor, but don't do any shuffle movement. Return to standing position, and then lower down for a body squat. Pull your arms wide keeping them parallel to the ground. Move your arms toward one another without crossing your hands, and then return as fast as you can (snake-like position).

Overhead Press Squat

This battle rope exercise is better than the conventional shoulder press. Stand with your feet a bit wider than the shoulder and grab the ropes on shoulder level. You need to make certain that there is enough tension in the ropes when you do with the basic shoulder press. Go down into a basic squat while pressing the ropes simultaneously overhead. Return to standing position.

Lateral Waves

Prepare your body to get moving with this battle rope exercise. Start by doing a basic alternating wave exercise. Start shuffling to one side, slamming the rope and shuffling about the same intensity. Once you are ready for the shuffle, lower down your body into a squat and then shuffle in the opposing side.

Chapter 4 - Increasing Strength and Endurance

Most experts in body training suggest that combining strength and endurance training can minimize the cardiovascular and muscular adaptations required to achieve optimum fitness. Similarly, adding aerobic exercises to a training program will limit the gains in strength and power as backed up by several studies done in the 1980s.

Hence, many athletes who need to build endurance usually avoid rigorous workouts for strength development. Strength training involves large numbers of repetitions and light weights. Ideally, you can use endurance training to improve short-term endurance and prevent muscle mass gains that could be an obstacle in achieving endurance for the long term.

But new research reveals that we need to re-consider the idea of mixing endurance and strength training. High-intensity strength training integrated with endurance exercises can actually provide benefits for better endurance while improving strength without considerable hypertrophy in the muscles.

Performing battle ropes exercises for strength and endurance can be an advantage for athletes who need endurance in the long term, as long as the workout is high intensity. Improved power, strength, and fitness could lead to better performance compared to endurance training only. However, athletes must exercise caution when using this type of battle rope program for young athletes and must avoid using it for pre-adolescent players.

Battle Ropes Exercises for Strength and Endurance

Lunge Jump Wave

Start with a battle rope alternating wave. Step right back for a reverse lunge, and then jump to switch legs so that you will land on the floor with your left leg. Repeat alternating legs smoothly and without losing form. Make sure that your chest and head is up during the entire exercise.

Jump Wave Squat

Mixed together, alternating waves and squats can be a total body exercise for strength and endurance, especially on the core. Do low alternating battle rope waves, and once the waves are constant, jump into the air and land in a full body squat. Repeat, and be sure to keep the wave stable during the entire movement.

180 Degrees Jumps

Face the anchor on your left side, and grab the ropes in each hand in front of your right hip with the palms opposing each other. Go down into a squat and jump into the air turning towards the direction of the anchor and rotate 180 degrees while swinging the rope overhead. Land smoothly in a full body squat, holding the ropes in front of the left hip. Repeat on the other side, and land bank in your first position.

Push-Up Wave Game

Start in a push-up position, holding one end of the rope in each hand. Do a knee tuck, return to push-up, immediately stand and do alternating waves for at least 15 seconds. Return to the push-up position, and then repeat.

Star Jumps

Begin by standing in a narrow squat and hold one end of the battling rope in each hand. Jump in the air and kick your legs to the sides. Swing your arms out the sides and overhead. Smoothly land in a squat position, placing your hand in front of your hips.

Chapter 5 - Nutrition

It is important to keep in mind that bodybuilding is about 50% nutrition. This is true, especially for novice athletes. Amateurs or those who are returning to the gym after quite some time can make considerable gains in mass, but not without proper nutrition. The more serious you are about muscle building, the more serious you should consider muscle gains.

Read the nine basic nutrition rules that every battle rope beginner must learn. Be sure to follow these rules and stick to the battle rope program for muscle gains, and soon you will see the results.

1. Patch Up on Protein

It is recommended to take at least one gram of protein for every pound of bodyweight every day. Protein is important in providing amino acids, which are used as the building blocks of muscle protein. Even though the recommended daily allowance for protein is set below half a gram for every pound of body weight for an average person, research reveals that athletes, particularly those who want to build mass and strength, should roughly double this recommended intake. Starters must actually try to take about 1.5 grams of protein for every pound of bodyweight every day for at least six months of doing battle ropes exercises, because this is when your muscles will react most rapidly to training. You can get proteins from turkey, fish, dairy, chicken, and beef.

2. Consume Carbs

Take about two to three grams of carbs for every pound of bodyweight every day. Carbs is the second most important macronutrient next to protein. They are stored in the muscles as glycogen and both keep the muscles full and large and provide a source of energy during training. For 180-pound starters, take at least 400 grams of carbs every day. Choose slow-digesting sources of carbohydrates such as oatmeal, fruits, vegetables, whole grains, beans, and sweet potatoes.

3. Don't Shy Away from Fats

At least 20% of your daily intake of calories should be sourced out from fat, and at least 5% of your fat calories must be saturated because high-fat diets will boost up your testosterone levels compared to low-fat diets. Maximizing levels of testosterone will improve muscle building without adding up layers of fat. Great sources of fats include ground beef, steak, mixed nuts, peanut butter, avocados, flaxseed oil, walnuts, salmon, catfish, trout, and olive oil.

4. Count Your Calories

For muscle gain, take at least 20 calories for every pound of bodyweight every day. It is important to take in more calories than your body can burn (positive calorie balance) to develop lean muscles. If you burn more calories than you take (negative calorie balance), your body will undergo conservation mode that doesn't support any muscle gain. Hence, a 180-pound athlete should get at least 3600 calories every day. Be sure that your calorie intake should first come from carbs (50%), protein (30%), and fat (20%).

5. Eat Often

It is best to take a meal that contains premium protein and carbs every two to three hours to ensure a stable supply of amino acids and energy for muscle gain for the entire day. This will help you gain mass and stay lean. Just make sure that every meal is about the same size. If you eat a heavy lunch, you will not be hungry for the next three hours and so you will gain weight, because excess calories will be stored as body fat. Take at least six meals every day for which starters should target at least 500 calories per meal.

6. Protein Shakes

Drink at least 20 grams of protein shakes before and after the workout. Basically, protein shakes are regarded as supplements, but they can be considered as important meals that you can consume at important times. Even though the diet must composed mostly of unprocessed foods, at times a protein shake can be a better choice, because you should not take complete meal at least 30 minutes before the workout. Instead, drink a 20-gram protein shake in order to prepare your muscle for the next session. Then at least one hour after the workout, drink another 20-gram protein shake.

7. Every Carb Has Its Time

Take a slow carb 30 minutes before doing any workout and primarily fast carbs after workout. As mentioned above, it is recommended to choose slower-burning carbs for most meals, including before the battle rope workout. Research reveals that when athletes consumer slow-burning carbs, they will have more energy and less fatigue during training but they can burn more fat while doing exercises and will not likely to experience hunger. Slow carbs include oatmeal, whole-grain bread, and fruits.

After battle rope workout, eat fast-burning carbs such as bagel, baked potato, and white bread. This will increase the level of anabolic hormone insulin that drives the carbs that you consume into muscle tissues, where they will be stored as glycogen that you can use for the next workout. Insulin is significant in driving amino acids into the muscle cells to develop muscle protein. This is also essential in driving creatine to the muscles and develops muscle protein synthesis - a major process by which muscle fibers grow. But be sure to control the level of insulin in the body for different health reasons.

8. Load Up Before Bed Time

Before sleeping at night, take at least 30 grams of casein protein shake or a cup of nonfat cottage cheese. Include two tablespoon of flaxseed oil, two tablespoons of peanut butter, or at least 2 ounces of mixed nuts. When we sleep, we are actually fasting for at least seven hours or depending on how long you sleep. Without food, the body tends to use amino acids stored in the muscle tissues to energize your brain. This is not a good thing if you want bigger and leaner muscles. The solution is not to sleep less but eat the right types of food before hitting the sack. Healthy fats and slow-burning proteins are highly recommended. These foods will help in slow digestion and supplying a steady source of amino acids for brain fuel, hence reducing the tendency of the body to use muscle.

9. Include Creatine in Your Diet

Add at least three grams of creatine with your protein shakes. Many body-building experts and scientists agree that creatine is great regardless of gender and age. Backed up by research, creatine is not only effective but also safe. Creatine usually comes in monohydrate form that when you take up could result to at least 10 pounds of lean muscle. It could also boost your strength and produce considerable endurance during the battle rope training.

Conclusion

Thank you for reading my book!

Battling ropes will help you to build muscle, lose weight, and increase strength and endurance. However, proper training is only 50% of the effort. To fully reap the rewards of the training, you need to ensure that your body is getting proper nutrition, and enough rest. It is also important to take note that consulting your doctor is crucial before trying any type of physical training. It is also recommended to consult a professional dietitian in planning your meals during the course of the battling rope workouts.

Bonus Content

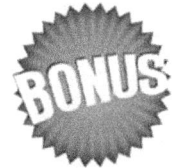

As a token of our appreciation Grand Reveur Publications would like to give you access to our exclusive bonus content (including free eBooks!).

Exclusive pre-release access to our latest eBooks Free Grand Reveur eBooks during promotional periods.

A method ANYONE can use to publish their own book and make passive income

To receive this bonus content visit the following web site:

https://ignorelimits.leadpages.net/grandreveur publications/

As this is a limited time offer it would be a shame to miss out, I recommend grabbing these bonuses before reading on.